DIABETES &
PREGNANCY:
WHAT TO EXPECT

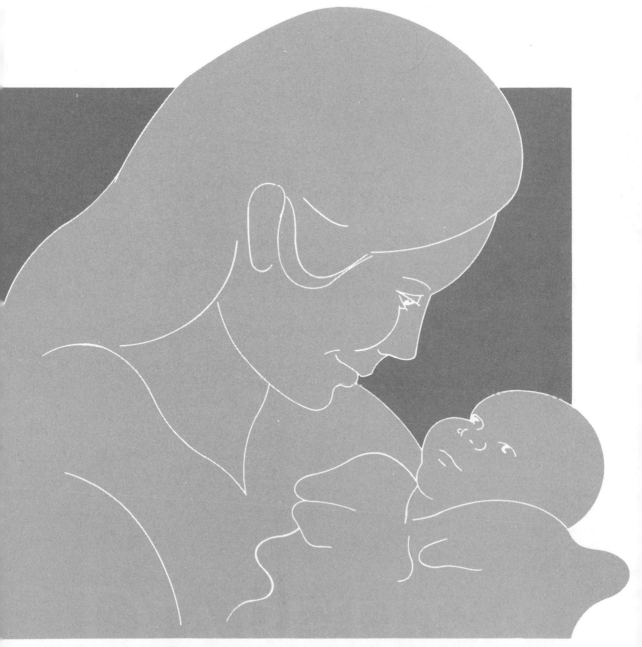

▲ ®American Diabetes Association ®

DIABETES & PREGNANCY:
WHAT TO EXPECT

Acknowledgments

This book was produced and written by members of the Task Force for the American Diabetes Association Council on Pregnancy. These members include: Lois Jovanovic-Peterson, M.D. (Chair); Nancy Cooper, R.D.; Marion Franz, R.D.; Priscilla Hollander, M.D.; Donald Coustan, M.D.; Robert Emling, M.S., Ed.D.; Lisa M. Fields, R.N., M.S.N.; Robin Goland, M.D.; John Hare, M.D.; Ronald Kalkhoff, M.D.; Deborah McCoy, R.N., M.S.; and Candace Wason, R.N., M.S.

We thank our reviewers for their time and expertise, including Pasquale J. Palumbo, M.D.; Steven G. Gabbe, M.D.; and Kathleen Wishner, Ph.D., M.D.

This book was produced with contributions from the staff of the American Diabetes Association National Center, in particular Craig D. Steinburg, Janice T. Radak, Susan H. Lau, and Caroline A. Stevens.

We are grateful to Lois Jovanovic-Peterson, M.D., for further reviewing this book for its second edition.

Table of Contents

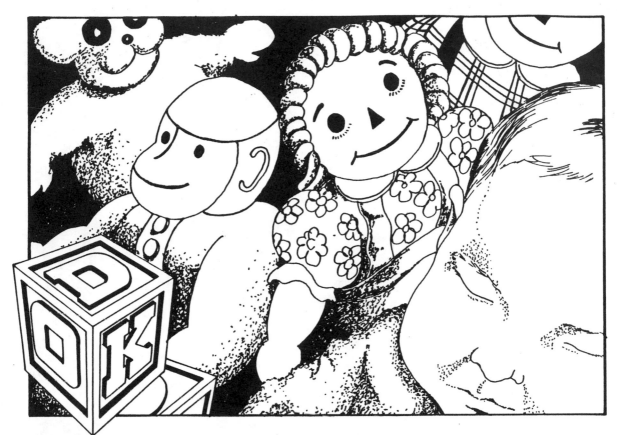

Introduction

Deciding to have a baby is one of the great decisions of your life. That one decision will result in numerous changes for at least the next 20 years: rattles, teddy bears, diapers, a crib; scuffed-up knees, toys in the driveway, kindergarten, back-to-school sales, school plays, the PTA; requests for the car, your permission, your approval, your wallet; college funds, fraternities, sororities, graduation parties; and more joy than you can imagine right now.

But, before all this takes place, you have to make the decision to do what it takes to give birth to a healthy, happy baby. And reading this book is the first step in making that decision.

CHAPTER 1

Diabetes, Pregnancy, and You

Y ou're reading this book because you're thinking about having a baby and you want to know more. You may have heard or been told that pregnancy is not for you because you have type I (insulin-dependent) diabetes. It is true that, in the past, pregnancy did present major problems for women with diabetes. But that's not the case today for most women.

Before insulin was introduced, women with diabetes rarely became pregnant, and if they did, their babies did not often survive. When insulin became available in the early 1920s, pregnancies became more common. Still, the number of successful pregnancies remained far below that of women who did not have diabetes.

The *good news* is that we now know that the key to a successful pregnancy for a woman with diabetes is tight blood-glucose control—both *before* conception and throughout pregnancy. Tight blood-glucose control means achieving a normal blood-sugar (glucose) level by testing blood glucose several times a day and properly balancing meals, exercise, and insulin. The goal of tight control is to keep blood-glucose levels as close to nondiabetic or "normal" as possible. With tight control and good obstetrical care, today the chances of having a successful pregnancy are almost the same as for a woman without diabetes. (Obstetrics is the medical specialty that deals with childbirth.)

Although the rate of successful pregnancies among women with diabetes has greatly improved, there are still some problems with which we need to be concerned. One problem is that the rate of birth defects in children born to women who have diabetes remains higher than among those born to nondiabetic women. Approximately 2 out of 100 normal (nondiabetic) pregnancies will result in babies with birth defects. For women who have diabetes, the range of birth defects is 2 to 23 percent and is dependent on the level of a woman's glucose control at the start of pregnancy.

Fortunately, however, we are learning how to increase the odds of producing healthy babies among women who have diabetes. We now know that many birth defects are related to the mother's blood-glucose control during the first eight weeks of pregnancy. This is because it is during this critical time that the baby's organs are formed. What is important to note here is that many women may not even know they are pregnant at this time.

The solution to the problem is obvious: *You must plan ahead for your pregnancy*. If you don't already practice good diabetes control regularly, your first priority should be to do so *before* you think further about having a baby. We suggest that a woman try to maintain good blood-glucose control three to six months *before* she plans to become pregnant. Of course, good control should be a lifelong practice.

It Takes Commitment

There has never been a better time for you, as a woman with type I diabetes, to plan for a pregnancy. By following a prescribed diabetes treatment program, you have a much better chance of giving birth to a healthy baby. But you will need to be committed to the work that pregnancy will take. It will certainly help if your partner is committed as well. This commitment should be based on a complete understanding of what is needed to achieve your goal. The fact that you're reading this book shows that you want to know more and that you care about your health and the health of your baby.

You will need and want a program of care that will help you obtain good blood-glucose control and will allow careful monitoring of your baby's progress. This program will require regular visits with your obstetrician and other members of your health-care team. The program will also include a variety of laboratory tests. It is possible that you might even be hospitalized for a time during your pregnancy—but only if problems arise.

Finally, care for women with diabetes during pregnancy is highly specialized. For this reason, you need a health-care team on your side. What is a health-care team? It is a group of health-care professionals who specialize in the different aspects of diabetes care. Your team could include the following:

- a physician or diabetologist who specializes in diabetes care and who is familiar with managing diabetes during pregnancy;
- an obstetrician who specializes in high-risk pregnancies and is experienced in managing pregnancies of women who have diabetes;
- a pediatrician or neonatologist who knows and can treat the special problems that can occur in a baby born of a woman who has diabetes;
- a registered dietitian who can adjust your meal plan to meet the needs you will have during your pregnancy;

■ and a diabetes nurse-specialist who can advise and teach you how to manage your diabetes.

Even with the help of these health-care professionals, following a good diabetes program during pregnancy won't be easy—it will take a lot of time and can sometimes be frustrating. It can also be expensive. However, all the time, energy, and effort can make all the difference in the health of your baby.

This book is designed to provide the information *you*—as a woman with type I (insulin-dependent) diabetes—need to have a successful pregnancy. (Editor's note: This book is specifically for the woman who has type I diabetes. From this point on, when we use the word "woman," we mean a woman who has type I diabetes.)

How Does The Team Approach Work?

Controlling diabetes is not always easy—even under the best of circumstances. It takes time and commitment on your part because you are ultimately responsible for your own health. Fortunately, though, you don't have to do it all alone. The American Diabetes Association recommends you use the health-care system to its fullest by using a "team approach" to diabetes care. A health-care team consists of experts in the different aspects of health care in general, and diabetes care in particular.

Each person's health-care team should meet his or her very personal health-care needs. Therefore, your team may include different health-care practitioners during different times in your life. Pregnancy is one such time.

The team approach helps your doctor provide you with expert care for all your specific needs. Diabetes care teams often include:

■ A diabetologist or physician who specializes in diabetes care and treatment. This person usually heads the health-care team as your primary source of care.

■ A nurse-practitioner, nurse-clinician, or nurse-educator. This is a registered nurse who has special clinical skills and can work with your physician in providing you with diabetes care. In addition, these nurses usually are trained to instruct and advise you how to manage your diabetes. Often, it is this individual you will deal with on the phone for routine management decisions or special sick-day procedures. You may check in with this particular member of your health-care team more often than the others.

- A registered dietitian. This person can help you design meal plans that meet your body's unique nutritional needs. As you grow older and your lifestyle and medical needs change, your diet will change as well. Your dietitian will be able to help you tailor your meal plans to reflect those changes.
- An eye doctor. This person can monitor the condition of your eyes and be on the guard for eye disorders that are common among people who have diabetes, such as retinopathy. The ADA recommends an eye examination when you decide to become pregnant and again when you become pregnant.
- A social worker or psychologist. This person can help you and your family members cope with any stress or anxieties that may come from learning to adjust to the diabetes lifestyle. These professionals can help you devise strategies for better relationships and teach you ways to reduce stress.
- An obstetrician who specializes in high-risk pregnancies and is experienced in managing pregnancies of women who have diabetes. This health-care professional is familiar with the extent of care that women wtih diabetes require when they become pregnant.
- A podiatrist (formerly called chiropodist). This health-care professional is trained to give proper care to your feet. Proper daily footcare is important for people with diabetes and should not be overlooked.
- A dentist who specializes in the care of your teeth. The ADA recommends that you have regular dental checkups.
- You, the individual with diabetes. You are the most important member of the health-care team because you call the shots. Like a quarterback on a football team, you must keep in touch with your health-care team to let them know how you are doing and whether you need help.

If you don't have a health-care team, your doctor may be a good source to help you find other health-care practitioners to meet your specific needs. Your local ADA affiliate or chapter may also be able to help. Many hospitals also have listings of health-care professionals.

The team approach was developed with people with diabetes in mind. It recognizes that people with diabetes are not sick; but rather, that people with diabetes require special guidance in maintaining their health.

Do not hesitate to contact your health-care practitioners when you have questions. Remember, they are there to help you.

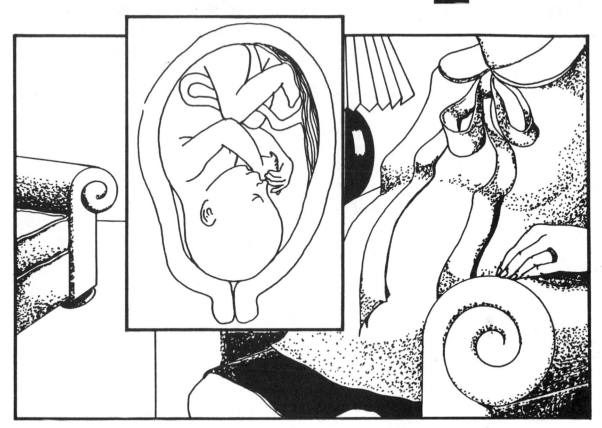

How Your Baby Develops

D uring the nine months that you are pregnant a lot of changes will take place. The end result of that pregnancy will change your life forever—you'll be a mother and at least partly responsible for the care of another human being. It's exciting, but still a big responsibility—one that really begins as soon as you become pregnant. In fact, it's possible that the most important care you ever give your child will be in those first few weeks of your pregnancy—a crucial time for the development of your baby.

Of course, each stage of your baby's development before he or she is born is important. And the best way to take care of your baby during this time is to take good care of yourself. If you are healthy, chances are good that your baby will be healthy, too.

Still, problems can occur. Finding problems and correcting them early are also important to the health of your baby. Numerous tests are available to help monitor and improve the success of your pregnancy. That's why regular checkups with your health-care team are so important during each month of your pregnancy.

CHAPTER 2

What To Expect in the Nine Months

A normal pregnancy lasts 40 weeks or about nine months. Pregnancy—technically known as gestation—is broken down into 3 three-month periods called *trimesters*. Each stage is exciting as your baby slowly develops and acquires all the physical characteristics he or she needs to live outside the womb. To give you an idea of your baby's progress, we will describe the different stages of development that normally occur during each trimester.

The first trimester In the first few weeks, your baby's heart forms and begins pumping blood. The digestive system, backbone, spinal cord, and brain begin to form. The placenta also develops during the first trimester. The placenta is the organ that surrounds your baby. Your baby receives nourishment through the placenta.

Around the eighth week, your baby will develop eyes (but the lids are still joined together), a nose, lips, and a tongue. Arms, elbows, forearms, hands, knees, lower legs, and feet begin to form. Before the ninth week, your baby was technically known as an *embryo*. But after the ninth week, it is called a *fetus*. (In this book, we will refer to a fetus as a baby.)

By the end of the first trimester your baby will be about 3 inches long and weigh about 1½ ounces. The buds and sockets for teeth in the jawbones begin to form. Fingernails and toenails start to develop, the earlobes are formed, and your baby will have most of his or her organs and tissues.

The second trimester Your baby continues to grow and develop. About a month into the second trimester (four months) your baby will weigh about 7 ounces and will be 6 to 7 inches long. Your baby's heartbeat will become strong and you may be able to hear it with either your doctor's stethoscope or the doppler device that amplifies the baby's heartbeat. The baby's muscles and bones are formed. Hair grows on the head and eyebrows begin to appear. And you may even feel the baby move!

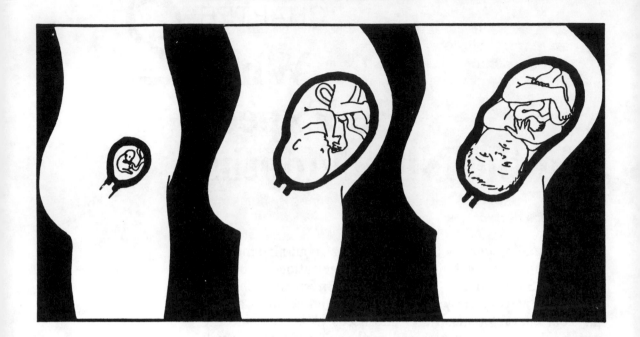

Near the end of the second trimester (six months) the baby will weigh close to 1¾ pounds and might be 11 to 14 inches long. You will notice your baby's movements more. The eyelids will separate and eyelashes will form. Also, the fingernails grow to the ends of the baby's fingers.

The third trimester All vital organs are fully formed. The baby's head bones are soft and flexible. Your baby will now begin to gain weight and grow rapidly. By the end of the seventh month, your baby will weigh 2½ to 3 pounds and be 14 to 17 inches long. By the time your baby is ready to be delivered, he or she will weigh about 7¼ to 7½ pounds and be close to 20 inches long.

Diabetes Control and a Healthy Baby

Each of these stages of gestation is important in your baby's development. And it is important that you keep your diabetes in control during each stage. It is *very* important that your diabetes be in control during conception and the first few weeks of the pregnancy. This is because the baby's vital organs (such as the heart, lungs, kidneys, and brain) are formed in the first weeks of gestation. So, a woman must seek care from her health-care team *before* she becomes pregnant.

Babies born to women with diabetes have a higher risk of birth defects than those born to women who don't have diabetes. Researchers suspect that poor diabetes control is at least partly responsible for these birth defects. Poor control of your diabetes—particularly in those early weeks—could expose your baby to high levels of glucose and ketones because both can pass through the placenta to the baby, but insulin cannot. The baby's exposure to higher than normal levels of glucose and ketones may increase the chances for birth defects (see Ketones, page 44).

These high levels of glucose can cause other problems for your little one in the last half of your pregnancy. When "fed" this extra glucose, a baby tends to get fat. Because the baby does not have diabetes, his or her pancreas will produce extra insulin to lower the blood glucose. So, the baby grows bigger and fatter than he or she would normally. This is sometimes called *macrosomia*.

A baby's production of extra insulin can cause another problem. It is hard to quickly stop the baby's pancreas from producing the extra insulin after he or she is born. So, the baby must go through a type of sugar *withdrawal* at birth.

During this withdrawal, the baby's blood-glucose level could drop dangerously low (hypoglycemia, see page 41). If hypoglycemia is not treated, it can cause serious problems for the newborn. Usually, the baby is given sugar through an intravenous line (IV) and is watched carefully for several days in the intensive-care unit of the hospital.

Another problem, called *jaundice*, is common among all babies but even more so among those born to women who have diabetes. Jaundice is a yellowing of the skin caused from a waste product. Before birth your baby needs a large supply of red blood cells. However, at birth your baby no longer needs this extra supply. So, after your baby is born, the baby's body will work through the liver to break down and excrete the old red blood cells. If your baby's liver isn't mature enough, it may have trouble handling this workload. Unfortunately, this creates a buildup of old red blood cells. The broken-down red blood cells or pigments are called *bilirubin*. Instead of being excreted, bilirubin is deposited in the baby's tissues. Bilirubin is what colors the skin yellow.

Babies born with jaundice are sometimes treated by being exposed to special lights. These lights help break down and get rid of bilirubin. In most children born with jaundice, this treatment is successful and lasts only a few days. But high levels of bilirubin can be toxic. If jaundice becomes severe enough, a baby might need a blood transfusion, but the chance of this happening is rare.

Another problem that rarely occurs and is not pleasant to discuss is stillbirth. Stillbirth happens when a baby dies before birth. Stillbirths used to occur more frequently among women with diabetes. But now, with expert care and good diabetes control, the chances for stillbirths are quite low. It may be necessary to deliver the baby a few weeks early to prevent problems, however.

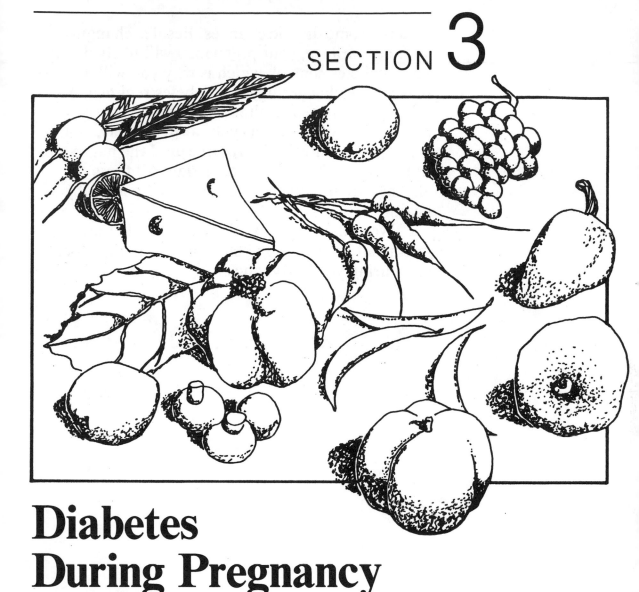

Diabetes During Pregnancy

Good diabetes control is important to your good health. And your unborn baby's health depends a lot on how healthy *you* are. So, good control plays a big role in the health of your unborn baby. If you are planning to have a baby, your diabetes should be in control *before* you become pregnant. This is because your baby will begin developing as soon as it is conceived—*before* you even know you are pregnant. And those first several weeks are crucial to your baby's development.

During your pregnancy, your body is going to

undergo some drastic changes. Besides changing your appearance, your pregnancy will likely disrupt your diabetes control, which is why you will need to make some changes in your diabetes regimen. You probably will need to alter the amount of insulin and number of injections you take each day, your meal plan, your exercise routine, and the number of times you test your blood each day. All these changes are designed to keep you and your baby healthy.

We will now discuss the elements that are important to managing your diabetes both before and during your pregnancy.

Insulin Therapy

D iabetes is a disease in which the body does not produce or respond to insulin (a hormone produced by the pancreas.) Without insulin, your body is unable to convert the food you eat into the energy you need to live, work, and play. Your body gets its energy from glucose, a form of sugar that is made from the food you digest. Insulin lowers blood-glucose levels by allowing the glucose to enter your body's cells. In other words, insulin acts as a key that unlocks the door to the cells to let glucose in. Only once it is inside those cells can glucose be used for energy. Without insulin, the glucose simply builds up in the bloodstream—a condition that is not healthy for your body.

Because you have type I (insulin-dependent) diabetes, you must inject insulin daily. (Insulin cannot be taken in pill form because your stomach juices would destroy its active materials before they had a chance to work.) Your insulin regimen—the combination of insulins and number of injections you will need—will be based on your body's special needs. As your baby grows, develops, and matures and as you change your schedule and your lifestyle, your insulin regimen will change too.

These changes or adjustments are just one part of the balancing act needed to maintain blood-glucose levels as close to normal as possible. *Normal* usually describes the blood-glucose levels of a person who does not have diabetes. In these individuals, fasting (or early morning) and pre-meal blood glucose should be 60 to 90 mg/dl. ("Mg/dl" means milligrams of glucose per deciliter of blood—a standard way of measuring blood-glucose levels.) About one hour after meals, your blood-glucose level should be below 140 mg/dl. And by two hours, it should be below 120 mg/dl. (In technical terms, these are called one-hour post-prandial and two-hour post-prandial levels or readings. These are general goals for pregnant women with diabetes; however, your individual blood-sugar goals must be worked out with your doctor or health-care practitioner.)

You will need to make these adjustments in your regimen because once insulin has been injected, it will work according to *its* action schedule—regardless of whether you follow yours! In other words, the insulin you injected before breakfast will start lowering your blood-glucose level as scheduled even if you didn't get to eat breakfast. So, working with your health-care practitioner to find an insulin regimen that suits your body's needs—as well as your lifestyle needs—is important.

Differences in Insulins

Many people are confused by the variety of available insulins and ask: Is there a difference? The answer is an overwhelming yes. Insulins vary in several ways. Years ago, the only kind of insulin available was animal insulin. Choices included either pork or beef insulin or a combination of the two. Today, human insulin is also on the market. This human insulin is chemically identical to that produced by a human pancreas, but it is made in the laboratory through a process called genetic engineering.

Insulins also vary in the timing of their action. There are three main types of insulin: Regular, also called rapid or short-acting; NPH and lente, also called intermediate-acting; and ultralente, also called long-acting. Regular insulins usually reach the bloodstream quickly (often within 30 minutes). This insulin is most effective (peaks) two to three hours after you inject it. It stays in your bloodstream about six hours—although not at full strength.

Intermediate-acting (NPH or lente) insulins take about four hours to reach your bloodstream. They peak seven to eight hours after injection; they can stay in the blood up to 18 hours.

Long-acting or *ultralente* insulins take four to six hours to reach your bloodstream. These insulins are strongest 14 to 18 hours after injection and can stay in the blood for up to 24 hours.

While your doctor or health-care practitioner will determine the exact combination of insulins you will use, the choice of how many injections you take and the method of insulin delivery depends on how easy it is to control your blood-glucose level. Chances are you will need a combination of insulins with different time actions, as well as several injections during the day.

There are several ways you can administer the insulin you need. Today's micro-fine needles make injections relatively painless. Some people choose jet injectors. These are mechanical devices that "shoot" the insulin through your skin in a jet stream. Still, others choose to use insulin pumps. Pumps are small, computerized devices that deliver insulin in a steady drip through a needle under the skin. However, the pump is not

Types of Insulin

	Source	Onset	Peak	Duration
Rapid Acting				
Humulin R (Lilly)	human	15-30 min.	hours 2-4	6-8 hours
Humulin BR (Lilly)	human	15-30 min.	hours 2-4	6-8 hours
Iletin I Regular (Lilly)	beef/pork	30 min.	hours 2-4	6-8 hours
Iletin II Regular (Lilly)	beef or pork	30 min.	hours 2-4	6-8 hours
Iletin I Semilente (Lilly)	beef/pork	1-2 hours	hours 3-8	10-16 hours
Velosulin-H (Novo-Nordisk)	human	30 min.	hours 1-3	8 hours
Velosulin-R (Novo-Nordisk)	pork	30 min.	hours 1-3	8 hours
Novolin R (Novo-Nordisk)	human	30 min.	hours 2½-5	6-8 hours
Purified Pork R (Novo-Nordisk)	pork	30 min.	hours 2½-5	8 hours
Purified Pork S (Novo-Nordisk)	pork	1½ hours	hours 5-10	16 hours
Regular (Novo-Nordisk)	pork or beef	30 min.	hours 2½-5	8 hours
Semilente (Novo-Nordisk)	beef	1½ hours	hours 5-10	16 hours
Novolin R Penfill (Novo-Nordisk)	human	30 min.	hours 2½-5	6-8 hours
Intermediate Acting				
Humulin L (Lilly)	human	1-3 hours	hours 6-12	18-24 hours
Humulin NPH (Lilly)	human	1-2 hours	hours 6-12	18-24 hours
Iletin I Lente (Lilly)	beef/pork	1-2 hours	hours 6-12	18-26 hours
Iletin II Lente (Lilly)	pork or beef	1-3 hours	hours 6-12	18-26 hours
Iletin I NPH (Lilly)	beef/pork	1-2 hours	hours 6-12	18-26 hours
Iletin II NPH (Lilly)	beef or pork	1-2 hours	hours 6-12	18-26 hours
Novolin L (Novo-Nordisk)	human	2½ hours	hours 7-15	22 hours
Novolin N (Novo-Nordisk)	human	1½ hours	hours 4-12	24 hours
Novolin NPH PenFill (Novo-Nordisk)	human	1½ hours	hours 4-12	24 hours
Long Acting				
Iletin I Ultralente (Lilly)	beef or pork	4-6 hours	hours 14-24	28-36 hours
Humulin U (Lilly)	human	4-6 hours	hours 8-20	24-28 hours
Ultralente (Novo-Nordisk)	beef	4 hours	hours 10-30	36 hours
Premixed				
Humulin 70/30 (Lilly)	human	30 min.	hours 2-12	24 hours
Novolin 70/30 (Novo-Nordisk)	human	30 min.	hours 2-12	24 hours
Novolin 70/30 PenFill (Novo-Nordisk)	human	30 min.	hours 2-12	24 hours
Mixtard (Novo-Nordisk)	pork	30 min.	hours 4-12	24 hours
Mixtard H 70/30 (Novo-Nordisk)	human	30 min.	hours 4-12	24 hours

Based on information from drug companies. Duration and peak actions may differ from one individual to the next.

recommended for everybody, and you must be highly motivated to use it. Discuss these options with your health-care team so that your decisions can be informed ones.

Insulin and Pregnancy

During your pregnancy, your body will go through some major changes. These changes will affect your blood-glucose level and make keeping your diabetes control difficult. One of

Estimated Action Times*

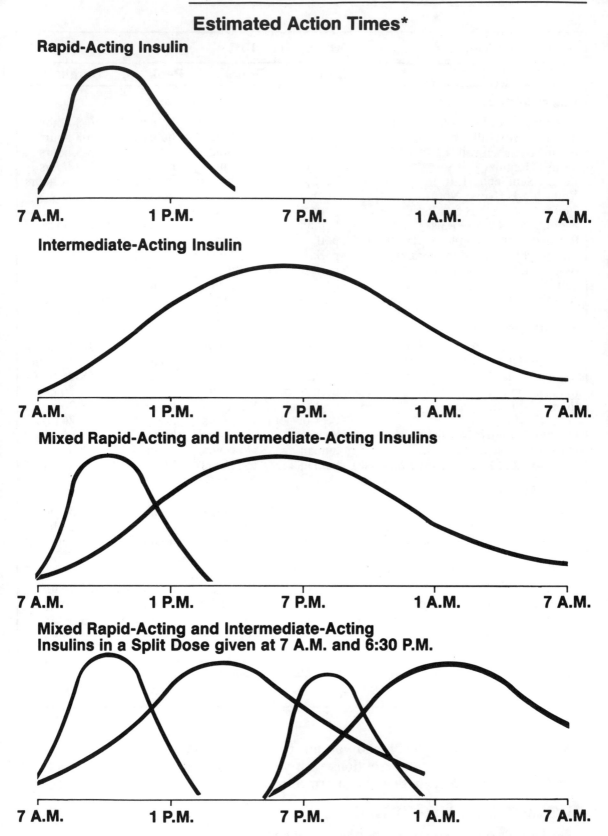

Rapid-Acting Insulin

7 A.M.   1 P.M.   7 P.M.   1 A.M.   7 A.M.

Intermediate-Acting Insulin

7 A.M.   1 P.M.   7 P.M.   1 A.M.   7 A.M.

Mixed Rapid-Acting and Intermediate-Acting Insulins

7 A.M.   1 P.M.   7 P.M.   1 A.M.   7 A.M.

**Mixed Rapid-Acting and Intermediate-Acting
Insulins in a Split Dose given at 7 A.M. and 6:30 P.M.**

7 A.M.   1 P.M.   7 P.M.   1 A.M.   7 A.M.

***Individuals respond to insulin at various rates; times presented here
are approximated. Chart assumes morning dose given at 7 A.M.**

the key changes in your diabetes care during pregnancy will be regular adjustments in your insulin program.

As your pregnancy progresses, your need for insulin will increase. This is because during pregnancy, the placenta produces hormones that decrease insulin's ability to lower blood glucose. Some women require double or even triple the amount of insulin they normally inject to maintain the same level of control. So, it's likely you will be put on an intensified insulin program. Like your usual insulin regimen, this intensified program may require that you increase your number of injections to three or four shots a day. The increase in insulin as well as the increase in the number of injections will help your body stay healthy while your baby is developing.

In addition to increasing your insulin program, your blood-testing regimen will probably intensify as well. (See blood-glucose monitoring, page 37.) Most women need to make changes in their insulin regimen about every 5 to 10 days because the need for insulin increases rapidly during pregnancy. Before and at different stages of your pregnancy, you will probably have a *hemoglobin A_{1C}* test (also known as a glycosylated hemoglobin test). This test is one way to measure your average blood-glucose control over the past six to eight weeks. Along with frequent blood testing, this test will help your doctor or health-care practitioner adjust your insulin regimen.

If you have questions, don't hesitate to ask a member of your health-care team for advice on how to make the necessary adjustments. You should *never* make changes without first checking.

CHAPTER 4

Nutrition, Diabetes, and Pregnancy

It is almost impossible to achieve good blood-glucose control without following a meal plan. This is because food raises your blood-glucose level. To keep your diabetes in control, you need to match the food you eat with the amount of insulin you inject and the exercise you do. So, it's important to be aware of not only *what* you eat, but also *how much* you eat, and *when* you eat it.

A dietitian or health-care professional with nutrition expertise will be able to help you design a meal plan especially for you. Your meal plan should include foods *you* prefer and meet *your* diabetes needs. Sound awful? Don't jump to conclusions—you may be surprised at how varied and flexible your meal plan can be.

In recent years, nutrition for people with diabetes has been examined and some changes have been made. People with diabetes are now encouraged to eat more complex carbohydrates, such as vegetables, breads, and pasta; more fiber; and less fat. You may even be able to eat small amounts of simple sugars (such as a small piece of unfrosted cake, a cookie, or a small scoop of ice cream) on special occasions—but check with *your* dietitian and doctor first so the appropriate exchange in food can be made, and, if necessary, your insulin dose can be raised. While it's true you won't be able to eat as freely as you did before your diabetes developed, you can still eat foods you enjoy.

Most people with diabetes have three meals a day and several well-timed snacks to make sure there is enough glucose in their blood at the time their insulin is peaking.

You don't have a meal plan? Don't worry. Instead, find a dietitian who can help you design one. If you don't know where to look, ask your health-care practitioner for help. Your hospital may also be a good resource. Or your local American Diabetes Association (ADA) affiliate may have a listing of dietitians in your area. (Check the white pages in the phone book for the number of an ADA affiliate in your area.)

Everyone, with or without diabetes, can benefit from meal planning—but this is especially true for mothers-to-be. That's because meal planning is based on the principles of good nutrition. And good nutrition is very important in having a healthy baby. Since it's so important, let's discuss what you need to do to meet the nutritional needs of you and your baby during pregnancy.

Meal Planning For a Healthy Baby

Much like preparing to run a race, you need to get yourself into condition before you become pregnant. Establishing good nutrition and eating habits before your pregnancy is a major part of *getting into condition*. This principle is true for all women considering pregnancy, but it is especially important for you because you have diabetes.

Of course, when it comes to good eating habits, you may be more fortunate than many women because you are probably more conscious of what you eat than those who don't have diabetes. In fact, women with diabetes often enter pregnancy with better nutritional habits than nondiabetic women!

Your nutritional needs change during pregnancy for two reasons. First, your baby needs nourishment. Second, your body will change the way it uses certain nutrients. It is important for you to practice good nutrition during pregnancy to fulfill the needs of your baby before birth as well as during lactation (breast-feeding). So let's begin by looking at the nutritional needs of your baby while he or she is developing and growing inside you.

Your Baby's Needs

People once thought that a developing baby could take whatever nourishment it needed from its mother. However, recent research has shown that this theory may not be true. Specifically, the growth and development of a baby is related to the mother's nutritional habits and weight gain. So, losing weight while you're pregnant is not recommended, but eating a well-balanced diet is. Here's why: When a mother doesn't get all the nutrients she needs—either because food is scarce or because she chooses not to eat enough—her supply of nutrients to her baby is reduced. The mother's body tries to protect itself from "starvation" *before* it protects the baby. This situation is particularly true in the second half of pregnancy. The consequences of poor nutrition may include health problems for the mother. It may also result in the birth of an underweight baby with nutritional, as well as other, deficiencies.

Poor nutrition can also affect the placenta, which performs several tasks essential to your baby's health. The placenta transports glucose, amino acids, hormones, and other substances from your body to your baby's system. If you are poorly nourished, the placenta cannot perform these functions properly.

So, good nutrition throughout pregnancy is important. Part of meeting your nutritional needs is making sure you gain enough weight over the nine months.

Weight Gain During Pregnancy

A weight gain of 22 to 32 pounds is considered appropriate for mothers who are at a normal weight when they become pregnant. However, this weight gain needs to be distributed properly. Just how much weight you will need to gain is a

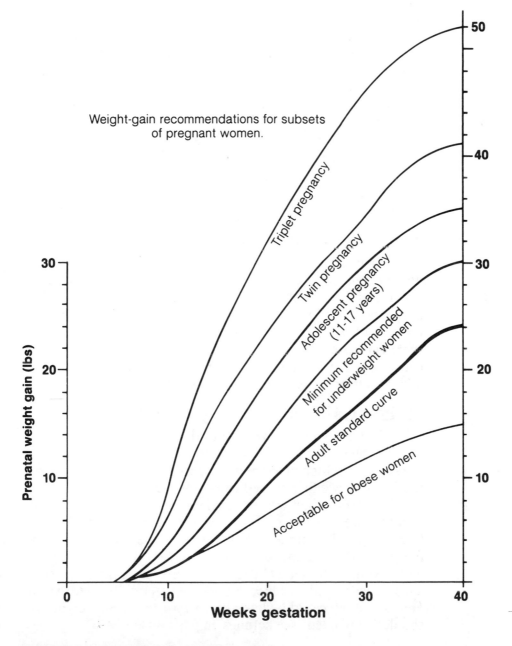

Weight-gain recommendations for subsets of pregnant women.

Triplet pregnancy

Twin pregnancy

Adolescent pregnancy (11-17 years)

Minimum recommended for underweight women

Adult standard curve

Acceptable for obese women

Prenatal weight gain (lbs)

Weeks gestation

determination your doctor or health-care practitioner will make, based on your body and your baby's needs.

The usual pattern of weight gain is quite small during the first three months—only about two to four pounds, unless you are underweight. If so, you will need to gain more. As your pregnancy progresses, you will need to gain more to assure adequate fat stores. Fat stores act as a reserve to provide for the added energy needs of you and your baby. In addition, they aid in providing nutrition during lactation. (If you are overweight, less of these fat stores will be needed.) During the second three-month period, you gain weight at a much faster rate—a little less than a pound a week on average. And during the last three months, the rate in which your body is gaining weight may slow down. Weight gains that follow the pattern we just mentioned have been shown to result in the best outcome of pregnancy. The figure on page 23 shows the different weight gain goals during pregnancy for various groups of women.

During pregnancy, it is more important to consider your pattern of weight gain rather than the total. If you start to gain a lot of weight suddenly or if you stop gaining weight or even start losing weight, your health-care team will want to know why. Any unusual changes in your weight should be discussed. If the problem is simply related to the food you eat, talk to your dietitian so that changes can be made in your meal plan.

Weight Gain For Underweight Mothers

About 10 percent of all women who become pregnant are underweight at the time of pregnancy. Another 10 percent become underweight because they do not eat properly during pregnancy. It is important to gain the proper weight to reduce the risk of having a baby with a low birthweight. However, there is no proof that forcing yourself to gain weight will also cause your baby to gain weight. How much should *you* gain? What your body needs to ensure a safe pregnancy.

Weight Gain For Overweight Mothers

Mothers who are overweight during pregnancy can also have problems, which may include: an increased incidence of *hypertension* (high blood pressure), and *preeclampsia* (hypertension and swelling caused from pregnancy).

If you have had weight problems before pregnancy, what should you know? First, pregnancy is definitely not a time to lose weight. The time to lose weight is before you become pregnant. If you don't eat enough calories during your pregnancy, your system may be forced to burn more fat than usual. This process will produce ketones and is called *starvation ketosis*, which could be harmful to your baby. So weight loss should be avoided (see ketones on page 44).

About 7 to 10 pounds of weight gain during pregnancy comes from an increase in fat stores. If before becoming pregnant you had extra fat stores, you may be able to gain less weight than the lean mother. How much weight *you* will need to gain will be determined by your doctor or health-care professional based on your nutritional needs and those of your unborn baby. In general, if you are obese, weight gain during pregnancy should probably be limited to 15 pounds.

Adolescents and Pregnancy

Teenagers who become pregnant need to gain more weight than most other women. Because her body is often still growing, a teen mother needs to provide for her body's own needs as well as for her baby's.

Distribution of Weight Gain

The figure below shows the average pattern of weight gain and the areas where weight gain occurs. You will notice that during the early part of pregnancy your baby will gain very little weight—not much more than 1 gram (about 1/28 of an ounce) of body weight per day. By contrast, your weight

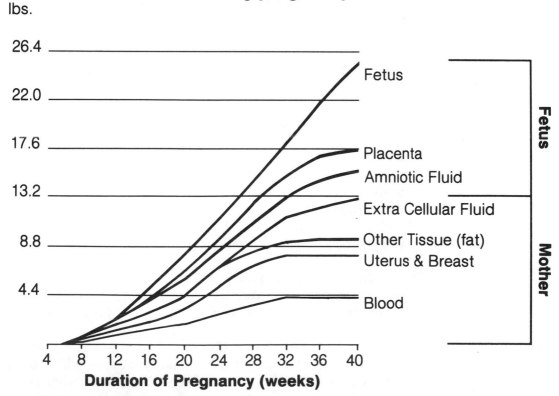

Breakdown of average weight gain during pregnancy

will increase rapidly during this time. Your uterus and breasts will enlarge, your blood volume will expand, and the placenta and amniotic fluid will be formed.

The fat stores in your body will increase rapidly in the early months. Around the fifth month or so, such storage will slow down. One of the first things you may notice when you become pregnant is a gradual thickening of your waist, back, and upper thighs. Don't be alarmed. This is natural and important. Your body is storing nutrients, so some reserves are available to safeguard the nutritional needs of your baby in the following months.

For the first four months, the daily nutrient needs of your baby are very small. However, by the sixth month your baby will gain approximately 10 times the weight each day that he or she gained early in pregnancy.

Calories Needed During Pregnancy

How many calories do you need during pregnancy to meet your weight goals? You need enough to provide your body with the energy it needs to function properly.

The best advice is to work closely with your dietitian to determine your calorie requirements. He or she will, with your help, determine a meal plan for you and your growing baby. Then, by monitoring your weight gain, you and your dietitian will know whether you are getting enough calories.

Nutrient Needs

Pregnancy has some very specific nutrient needs. A discussion of some of the nutrients you need during your pregnancy follows.

Protein Protein—largely derived from meat and milk products—is abundant in North American diets. Protein during pregnancy helps to expand your blood volume and growth of breast and uterine tissues. However, the diets of most women already include plenty of protein to meet these needs. This is especially true if you have diabetes. In most cases, if you add two glasses of skim milk to your prepregnancy meal plan, you can be sure you are eating adequate amounts of protein.

Iron You need more iron while you are pregnant for two reasons: to provide for your increased production of blood, and to supply iron to your unborn baby, so he or she can produce blood.

Iron from your diet is also stored by your baby in his or her liver. If your diet is rich in iron, then your baby will be born with enough iron stores to last through the months when he or she is mainly fed milk. (Milk, unless fortified, does not contain iron.) Most foods don't contain enough iron for you to get what you need. So, unless you are willing to eat liver once or twice a week, you will likely be asked to take an iron supplement.

Folic Acid   You will need almost double the usual amount of folic acid during pregnancy. It is possible for you to get the folic acid you need from food since this vitamin is widely distributed in common foods. Some good sources are dark green leafy vegetables like spinach and kale, dried beans, liver, oranges, and whole-wheat products.

Folic acid forms co-enzymes, which are needed for rapid cell division, such as occurs during pregnancy. Folic acid is also essential for the formation of red blood cells in both you and your baby.

Calcium   Calcium is another nutrient needed in larger amounts during pregnancy. Calcium is important to bone development and strength. Milk is a good source of calcium and a daily intake of 1,200 mg is recommended. One quart of milk or the equivalent in other milk products will meet your calcium requirements. Vitamin D is important along with calcium because it promotes calcium absorption. You can get a sufficient amount of calcium by drinking vitamin D-fortified milk and through exposure of the skin to sunlight. If you are allergic to milk, you may need to take a calcium supplement, preferably calcium carbonate. Ask your doctor or dietitian about calcium supplements.

Vitamin Supplements   Eating a well-balanced diet will usually provide the vitamins and minerals you need while pregnant. However, you may not get the amount of iron and folic acid you and your baby need. For this reason, you may have to take vitamin supplements.

The need for other vitamins (such as the B vitamins or vitamin C) increases only slightly during pregnancy. Very large amounts of some vitamins can be harmful to both you and your baby. Therefore, large doses (amounts greater than 100 percent of the Recommended Dietary Allowance) of vitamins and minerals should be avoided.

Sodium   In the past, sodium was restricted, but we now know that it is necessary during pregnancy. You do not need to increase sodium intake, since you are probably consuming enough already.

Caffeine   Caffeine is a colorless, bitter substance that works as a stimulant (increases the activity) for the heart and central nervous system. It is found in coffee, tea, and many carbonated beverages. The danger of caffeine to the developing baby has been studied mostly in animals. These studies show some behavioral changes and problems in growth in animals exposed to caffeine. Studies in humans are very limited. However, in 1981, the U.S. Food and Drug Administration issued a general warning encouraging women to avoid unnecessary consumption of caffeine during pregnancy. So, it's probably a good idea for pregnant women who choose to use caffeine to do so in moderation. (What is moderation for you may not be the same for another woman. Ask your health-care practitioner how much caffeine would be safe for you.)

Saccharin and Aspartame   Mothers with diabetes are often concerned about the safety of using artificial sweeteners, such as saccharin and aspartame (Equal® or NutraSweet®), during pregnancy. We do know that saccharin can cross the placenta to the baby, but no one is sure whether this transfer is a problem. So, we recommend that saccharin be avoided during pregnancy.

Aspartame is composed of *aspartate* and *phenylalanine*. Aspartate seems to cause little concern for pregnant women because it does not cross the placenta. Phenylalanine does cross the placenta, but it seems unlikely that an average intake (such as two or three soft drinks a day) could raise the level close to a dangerous level.

Alcohol   Today, we know that it can be dangerous to drink alcohol during pregnancy. *Fetal alcohol syndrome*, which occurs in infants born to mothers who drink alcohol regularly, can cause birth defects such as unusual facial characteristics, low birth weight, and defects in the baby's central nervous system that might result in a decrease in intellectual abilities, perhaps even mental retardation.

It appears that even low doses of alcohol—such as two beers a night—if consumed regularly by the mother, may result in growth failure and/or lower IQ in her baby. Moderate amounts of alcohol appear to double the risk of a miscarriage, as well as growth failure of the baby. No one knows whether there is a safe level of alcohol during pregnancy.

The best advice for pregnant women is to abstain from alcohol use altogether. It may also be wise to abstain if you are trying to conceive.

Smoking   Cigarette smoking can lead to having an infant with a low birth weight. In contrast to alcohol, most of the growth retardation caused by smoking occurs during the last three months of pregnancy. Stopping smoking even as late as the last few months will reduce its harmful effect. Smoking will not affect *your* weight gain but can affect your baby's.

The more a mother smokes, the higher her risk for problems. So, if you can't stop smoking, you should at least try to cut back on the number of cigarettes you smoke. The earlier a mother stops smoking, and the less she smokes, the better.

Cocaine and Other Drugs   While you are pregnant, it is very important that you use only those medications specifically prescribed for you. While the so-called "recreational drugs," such as cocaine, are harmful for you at any time, using these drugs during your pregnancy can result in harmful effects for your baby. Some of the problems that can result include: birth of an underweight and undersized baby, mental retardation, and *abruption* (a life-threatening condition for the baby). The best advice is to abstain from any harmful drugs completely.

Nutritional Issues Related to Diabetes

Mothers with insulin-dependent diabetes have additional concerns about nutrition during pregnancy. These include keeping blood glucose within "normal" ranges during this nine-month period.

To keep blood glucose in line, you will need to stick to your pregnancy meal plan throughout the day. The balancing of food and insulin will help prevent hypoglycemia (low blood glucose, also known as an insulin reaction) and hyperglycemia (high blood glucose).

The importance of eating these regular meals and snacks cannot be emphasized enough. Women often respond to an occasional high blood-glucose level by skipping a meal or snack, especially at night. However, you need to remember that blood-glucose values reflect what has happened during the *previous* one to three hours. When you eat, you are eating to prevent hypoglycemia during the *next* two to three hours.

If you find that your blood glucose is always high at certain times of the day, call your doctor or health-care practitioner to help you make the proper adjustments in your insulin regimen or meal plan.

Bedtime snacks are especially important during pregnancy. Your baby feeds from your supply of glucose 24 hours a day, not just during the 12 hours when you are awake and eating. As a result, overnight insulin reactions are common. Your evening snack should probably include foods containing all three nutrients—protein, carbohydrate, and fat. Milk and other dairy products are a good example. Some women find they even need to eat during the middle of the night. Often, a glass of milk (8 ounces) during the night is enough to prevent the blood glucose from dropping too low.

During the first three months, you may find you are eating less (and so taking in fewer calories) than you were before you were pregnant. This is especially true if you are nauseated because of morning sickness. As you get over that period, you will probably want to eat more to meet your increasing calorie needs.

How you distribute calories throughout the day is important. Three meals and three snacks are usually recommended. Breakfast is likely to be your smallest meal because blood-glucose values are frequently highest in the morning. Blood-glucose monitoring can help you and your dietitian schedule your meal plan correctly.

Problems with Pregnancy

Nausea and Vomiting   Try the following for nausea:
- Eat crackers or dry toast when you wake up and before you get out of bed. (Although no research has demonstrated why this helps, it may be related to a low blood-glucose level. Remember, these foods are pure carbohydrate, so your morning insulin dose will have to be adjusted to accommodate these foods.)
- Eat smaller meals and eat more often.
- Drink fluids between meals instead of with meals.
- Avoid spicy and greasy foods.
- Avoid lying down right after eating.

Constipation   Constipation is common during pregnancy. One reason is because your intestinal muscles become more relaxed. Another reason is that your growing baby puts more pressure on your intestines. If you have problems, try the following:
- Drink plenty of liquids.
- Eat high-fiber foods, including whole-grain breads, bran cereal, raw fruits, and vegetables.
- Get plenty of exercise.
- If the problem persists, discuss it with your health-care practitioner.

Heartburn   As your pregnancy progresses, you may get heartburn. Some symptoms of heartburn include burning discomfort in the stomach or throat, an upset stomach, or a stomachache. The following may help:
- Eat frequent, small meals.
- Avoid greasy or spicy foods.
- Eat slowly, being sure to chew food well.
- If heartburn persists, check with your doctor for help.

Cravings   At some stage in pregnancy many women find that their food likes and dislikes change. During their pregnancy, some women may dislike foods they normally like. At the same time, they may have a craving for foods they normally would not eat. So, you may need to make changes in your meal plan to fit your new likes and dislikes. Your dietitian will work with you.

Medications   Since many medications can be harmful to your baby, avoid all medications except those prescribed for you during your pregnancy. Check with your doctor before using any over-the-counter medications.

CHAPTER 5

Exercise, Diabetes, and Pregnancy

Physical activity can be good for you—especially when you have diabetes—because in most cases exercise will lower your blood-glucose level. Exercise is also helpful in losing weight, which is a concern for many people who have diabetes. (Caution: Do not attempt to lose weight while you are pregnant unless you are under a health professional's care.) Exercise can also help improve your muscle tone, circulation, and heart function. Finally, exercise is beneficial because it can give you a feeling of well-being.

All women are unique, and some are more fit than others. Some are able to run marathons, while others have conditions that prevent them from doing any strenuous exercise. So, it is important to find a level of exercise that's safe for you— before, during, and after pregnancy. Exercise can be beneficial, but only when it is done correctly and at a safe level. Be sure to discuss an exercise program with your doctor before you start. Your doctor needs to check the condition of such things as your eyes, blood pressure, and heart. These checkups are important to be sure you are physically fit to exercise and to see whether your body can handle an exercise program as it adjusts to the stress of pregnancy. When you become pregnant, you should discuss any changes that may need to be made in your exercise program as your pregnancy progresses.

Finding a good exercise program is not the only thing you will need to be concerned with. Besides the struggle you may have just getting the ambition to exercise, you need to think about how your exercise will affect your diabetes. In most cases, exercise lowers blood glucose. Therefore, whenever you exercise, it is important to monitor your blood-glucose level. This means testing your blood before and after you exercise. (If your blood-glucose level is 240 mg/dl or above, you should not exercise. When your glucose level is this high, exercise may only raise it higher. And when you are pregnant, if your blood-glucose level reaches 240 mg/dl, you should contact your practitioner immediately.)

Monitoring your diabetes also means learning to recognize the symptoms of an insulin reaction (low blood glucose, see hypoglycemia, page 41) during and after you exercise. To help avoid an insulin reaction, it is important to coordinate your exercise program with your meals and with the timing and amount of insulin you inject. If you exercise more or less than planned or at a different time, you may upset your blood-glucose level. Your health-care team will be able to help you work your exercise program into your diabetes regimen.

If you feel a reaction coming on while you are exercising, *stop* and treat it with some form of sugar. Things you could treat a reaction with are: 4 ounces of orange juice, 2 or 3 pieces of hard candy, 4 ounces of a nondiet soft drink, or 2 glucose tablets. Ask your dietitian for other choices that you can treat an insulin reaction with. Once you feel better, you should eat some protein, such as half a meat sandwich, a piece of cheese, or a glass of milk.

By working closely with your health-care team, carefully monitoring blood glucose, balancing food and insulin, and participating at an appropriate level of exercise, you should be able to maintain a good level of diabetes control. Be smart and take the time to prepare properly for any exercise routine. Also, be careful not to overdo it—too much exercise too soon can be harmful for anyone.

Exercise and Pregnancy

You may already be a part of a growing number of women who are regularly involved in exercise programs. Like many of these women, you may have concerns about whether you can continue your exercise routine after you become pregnant. Because you have diabetes, you likely have questions about how exercise will affect your blood-glucose control during pregnancy.

In the past, pregnant women with diabetes were advised not to exercise because many people feared exercise would affect the health of the baby. Today, however, women who have regularly exercised before pregnancy can often continue exercising during pregnancy. Of course, they may need to exercise at a more moderate level while they are pregnant. If you have not been involved in regular exercise, you should not start a strenuous exercise program while you are pregnant. Whether you have been exercising or not, there may be some exercises that you won't be able to do while you're pregnant.

Exercises you may be excluded from include such things as racquet sports, golf, volleyball, and basketball. These activities involve twists, turns, jumping, and sudden starts and stops—all of which can strain your muscles, joints, and ligaments and have a harmful effect on your baby. You should also avoid hazardous activities such as water and snow skiing. (The

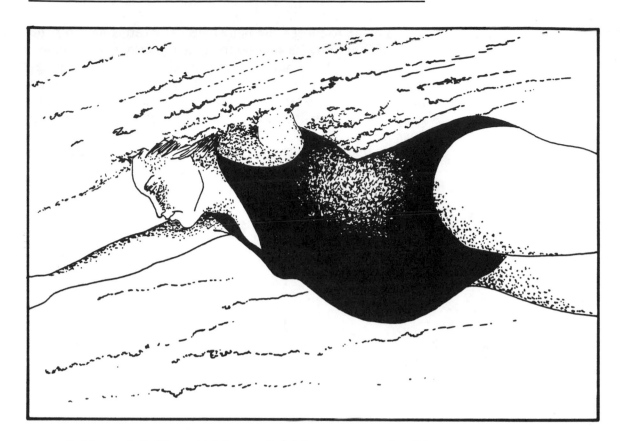

potential harm is falling at high speeds.) Many women should also avoid jogging while pregnant. (Falling is a concern, but the pounding could prove harmful to your pregnancy.)

While you may have to eliminate some activities while you are pregnant, there are other exercises you can do to stay fit. For example, brisk walking may be a good alternative. Many people who found jogging too strenuous have benefited from walking. A brisk walk after a meal may be ideal for controlling your diabetes. This may be especially true after breakfast, since many times blood-glucose levels are highest in the morning.

Swimming can also be good exercise for many women who are pregnant. It isn't bone-jarring or hard on your feet and legs and the buoyancy of the water eases stress on your joints. Thus, you are freer from injuries. Some areas offer *water aerobics* classes.

You may also be able to participate in an aerobics program, but at a lower level than you may be used to. A good alternative may be low-impact aerobics. This method allows you to get an aerobic workout but is designed to lessen the impact on your body.

Postnatal Exercises

Remember, the need for fitness never stops—not even during the excitement of caring for your baby and rescheduling your life to meet your baby's needs. Exercising after the birth of your baby is essential to good diabetes control. It will also help your body make the major adjustments after pregnancy. Toning your muscles helps your body "shrink" to the firm shape it was before you were pregnant. If you don't exercise, you may find it much harder to tighten your body up later.

You can probably start exercising four to six weeks after your baby is born. If you have a cesarean section, you may have to wait a little longer. Ask your health-care practitioner when you can safely return to your prepregnancy exercise program.

Monitoring 6 Your Diabetes

T o know how well you are controlling your diabetes, you are going to have to test your blood and your urine. These tests will help you make the needed adjustments to keep your diabetes control on target. This chapter explains blood-glucose monitoring and urine tests and the role each plays in your diabetes control.

Blood-Glucose Monitoring

In the early 1980s, self-monitoring of blood glucose became available. This *method* has made it possible for you to test your blood glucose anywhere you choose. This advance has contributed greatly to diabetes management—and has increased your chances of having a successful pregnancy as well.

Of course, if you test your blood but fail to make needed adjustments in your diabetes regimen, blood testing won't do you any good. It is important that you record the results of each test so that you and your health-care team can see how well your diabetes regimen is helping to control your diabetes and can make changes, if needed.

There are two ways to test your blood. In both, you first prick your finger with a special needle called a lancet to get a drop of blood. You then place the drop of blood on a test strip. The steps you follow to do your blood test will depend on what type of test strip you use or what type of meter you use. Ask your doctor or health-care practitioner walk through the testing process you need to follow.

In one method, you wait for the test strip to change colors. (The glucose causes the change.) You then match the color of the strip to a color chart, which is usually on the test strip container. The colors represent *ranges* of glucose levels, such as 60 to 90 mg/dl. If your test strip colors match those colors, then your blood-glucose level falls somewhere in that range.

In the second method, you place the test strip in a blood-glucose meter. A meter is a small computerized machine that "reads" your test strip. Your blood-glucose level is displayed on a digital screen (like that of a pocket calculator).

Meters provide more accurate blood-glucose readings than matching the test strip colors to a chart. This is because meters give you an exact number instead of an estimate or range of your blood-glucose level. And as you prepare for pregnancy or if you are pregnant, accuracy is extremely important. For someone who is visually impaired or color blind, a meter is essential.

Most people with diabetes are now advised to test their blood glucose four times a day as a way of tracking diabetes control. Generally, tests are done before breakfast, lunch, and dinner and at bedtime. During your pregnancy, you may be asked to test after your meals or even during the night. Testing regimens, like insulin therapy, are individually tailored to each woman and her pregnancy.

Urine Tests

Before blood-glucose monitoring became available, urine tests were the only way a person could monitor diabetes control. But now, because of blood-glucose testing, most people test their blood rather than their urine to monitor diabetes control. That's because urine tests are much less accurate— they can only give you an estimate of your glucose level at the time of the test. In fact, the "reading" from a urine test may actually show what your glucose level was hours before the test rather than what it actually is. Such an estimate will not provide you with the information you need to maintain good or tight diabetes control.

Still, urine tests do provide vital information that will help you detect *ketoacidosis*. In fact, testing your urine is the only way to measure ketones (see ketones, page 44). Ketones are bad for your health and your baby's. While you are pregnant, you are at a higher risk for developing ketones. So, you may be asked to test your urine for ketones more than you did before you were pregnant.

Urine tests are fairly easy to do. First, you take a sample of your urine and place a test strip in the sample. Like the blood-glucose strips, this strip will change color. You match the color to a chart, which will give you an indication or range of the amount of ketones present in your urine. If your urine test detects ketones, you should contact your health-care practitioner.

Making Adjustments

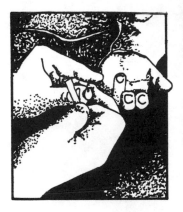

As you work to control your diabetes, it's likely you'll need to make adjustments occasionally—some major ones, some minor ones. You may have to change your meal plan, your exercise routine, or insulin dosage—or possibly all three because of the changes your body makes during pregnancy. For example, most women need to make changes in their insulin regimen about every 5 to 10 days because the need for insulin increases rapidly during pregnancy. Other things may make it necessary to make adjustments. For example, you may change jobs, have a different work schedule, or become more active. Sometimes you have to make sudden adjustments because of changes in your daily routine, such as an unexpected physical activity. Sometimes your diabetes regimen is just not working to control your diabetes. The important thing to remember is not to feel you are stuck with a certain diabetes program. If you are having trouble controlling your diabetes, adjustments will need to be made. Members of your health-care team can help you set up guidelines on how to change your diabetes regimen when needed. You should never make changes without first checking with your doctor or health-care practitioner.

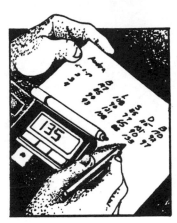

Recording the results of your blood-glucose tests and urine tests is important because this information is vital to making adjustments in your diabetes regimen. As you and your health-care team work together, you should be able to find an insulin regimen that will work to keep you healthy.

CHAPTER 7

Problems Associated With Diabetes

It would be wonderful if practicing good diabetes control would eliminate all the difficulties that relate to diabetes. Unfortunately, it just isn't so. While you have a better chance of preventing any problems by adhering to your diabetes regimen, you will still experience occasional problems with such things as hypoglycemia, hyperglycemia, and ketones. The trick is detecting these problems early and treating them before they get worse. If left untreated, these problems can have serious consequences for you and your baby. That's why we've chosen to discuss each in more detail.

Hypoglycemia

Hypoglycemia is low blood sugar. It is sometimes called an insulin reaction. An insulin reaction can be caused by a number of things: You may have taken too large a dose of insulin, eaten too little food or not eaten on time, or exercised too much.

Testing your blood is the best way to know whether your blood glucose is low. But, there are other symptoms that will help you recognize an insulin reaction. The symptoms include:
- shakiness or dizziness
- sweating
- clumsy or jerky movements
- hunger
- headache
- sudden moodiness or behavior changes, such as crying for no apparent reason
- pale skin color
- difficulty paying attention or confusion
- tingling sensations around the mouth

If you experience these symptoms, you should test your blood sugar. If it is low, treat it immediately. If you can't test, you should treat the reaction. It is better to have too much sugar than to suffer a severe insulin reaction.

You can treat a reaction by eating or drinking some form of sugar. Some examples would be: 3 to 4 pieces of hard candy

Symptoms of Hypoglycemia

- shakiness or dizziness
- sweating
- clumsy or jerky movements
- hunger
- headache
- sudden moodiness or behavior changes, such as crying for no apparent reason
- pale skin color
- difficulty paying attention or confusion
- tingling sensations around the mouth

or sugar cubes, 4 ounces of orange juice, 4 ounces of a nondiet cola drink, or 2 glucose tablets. About 20 minutes after you treat an insulin reaction, you should test again—just to be sure your blood-glucose level has risen. If it hasn't, you may need to eat more. After you feel better, eat some protein, such as a couple pieces of cheese, half a sandwich, or 8 ounces of milk. Such instances should always be recorded in a notebook because your health-care team will need to know about them.

Note: These are only suggestions. You should check with your dietitian for specific ways to treat a reaction. Also, your dietitian may suggest alternatives to treating an insulin reaction during your pregnancy.

Hypoglycemia is always a potential problem for a person with diabetes, but it can be particularly so during pregnancy. This is because hypoglycemia can occur more rapidly and without the usual warning signs. To avoid problems, we recommend testing blood glucose when insulin is peaking, or most effective. For example, if you inject Regular insulin at 7:30 a.m. and eat your normal meal as scheduled, your insulin would be most effective about three hours later. So, you would want to check your blood-glucose level between 10 and 10:30 a.m. If your blood-glucose level was below 60 mg/dl, you would most likely increase your morning snack according to the instructions of your health-care practitioner, or decrease your usual morning insulin dose.

You should always be prepared to treat hypoglycemia, but especially when you're pregnant. To be safe, you should have a *glucagon kit* in your home and at work for severe cases of hypoglycemia. Glucagon is a hormone that causes your blood sugar to rise. It is used primarily to treat someone who has passed out from hypoglycemia. It is a good idea to teach family members and co-workers how and when to inject glucagon, just in case a severe reaction should happen to you. A member of your health-care team can teach you how to use glucagon.

Signs and Symptoms of Hyperglycemia

- high blood sugar
- high levels of sugar in the urine
- frequent urination
- increased thirst
- headaches
- tiredness and fatigue

Hyperglycemia

Another problem that accompanies diabetes is *hyperglycemia*. Hyperglycemia is high blood sugar. It happens when your body has too little, or not enough, insulin, or when too much food is eaten.

Hyperglycemia can happen for several reasons. You may eat more than you planned or exercise less than planned. Other things can cause hyperglycemia such as the stress of an illness, such as a cold or the flu. Or emotional stresses, such as family or work conflicts.

The signs and symptoms of hyperglycemia include:

- high blood sugar
- high levels of sugar in the urine
- frequent urination
- increased thirst
- headaches
- tiredness and fatigue

Like *hypo*glycemia, the best way to avoid *hyper*glycemia is to test your blood regularly and then treat high blood sugar early before other symptoms appear. Your doctor can tell you what level is considered high. Generally a blood-glucose level of 140 mg/dl or above is considered high during pregnancy.

If you do not treat hyperglycemia, a condition called ketoacidosis (diabetic coma) could occur. Ketoacidosis happens when your body has too many ketones (see ketones, page 44). Ketoacidosis is life-threatening and needs immediate treatment.

How do you treat hyperglycemia? There are three ways to lower blood-glucose levels—exercise, eat less food, take more insulin. The method you use will depend on the circumstances at the time of the high blood-glucose reading. You and your health-care practitioners need to work out procedures for handling one-time instances of hyperglycemia as well as more detailed instructions for handling patterns of hyperglycemia. Exercise is often the first method used to lower blood glucose. If this does not work, you may be asked to eat less at a given meal or snack. Finally, you may have to change the amount of insulin you inject or the timing of the injections. Your practitioners should be able to help you find the best way to lower your blood glucose. You should not change your diabetes regimen without first checking with your health-care team. (And if your blood glucose is 240 mg/dl or above, you should not exercise. If you are pregnant and your blood glucose tops 240 mg/dl, call your health-care practitioner for immediate help. Blood-glucose levels this high may be harmful to your baby.)

How will hyperglycemia affect your health or the health of your baby while you are pregnant? If your diabetes is not in control during the early part of your pregnancy, you increase the risk of having a baby with birth defects.

Hyperglycemia also increases the chance of having a large baby who may go through a "sugar withdrawal" at birth. In a sense, your baby may become "addicted" to your high blood sugar. This means that once the baby is born, he or she may become severely hypoglycemic because the level of blood sugar is not as high as he or she was getting inside of you. This condition could cause the baby to have seizures. Also, a large baby increases the risk that you will have your baby by cesarean section (see page 51).

Warning Signs of Ketoacidosis

- **a dry mouth**
- **thirst (but not hunger)**
- **nausea**
- **excessive urination**
- **dry skin**
- **fruity-smelling breath**
- **abdominal pain**
- **vomiting**
- **if advanced, unconsciousness**

Testing for Ketones

Ketones are acid substances that are produced when the body breaks down fats because no other source of energy is available. This process happens when there is not enough insulin to let glucose (the main source of energy) enter the cells and provide the body with the energy it needs. Your body cannot tolerate large amounts of ketones and will try to get rid of them through the urine. Unfortunately, your body cannot get rid of all the ketones, so they build up in your blood.

Of course, small amounts of ketones in the morning are not uncommon during pregnancy. Check with your doctor for the specifics of how you should handle this condition. You should test your urine for ketones whenever your blood glucose is greater than 200 mg/dl (see urine testing, page 38). Ask when and how often you should test for ketones—especially while you are pregnant.

If ketones continue to build up in the blood a condition called ketoacidosis could happen. Ketoacidosis is the name of the condition in which you have too many ketones. Ketoacidosis can be life-threatening and needs immediate treatment. Different from insulin reactions, ketoacidosis usually develops gradually over many hours.

There are several warning signs of ketoacidosis:

- a dry mouth
- thirst (but not hunger)
- nausea
- excessive urination
- dry skin
- fruity-smelling breath
- abdominal pain
- vomiting
- if advanced, unconsciousness

Whenever you detect any of these symptoms, you should contact your health-care practitioner. Usually, ketoacidosis must be treated in the hospital, where fluids can be restored and diabetes can be brought under control.

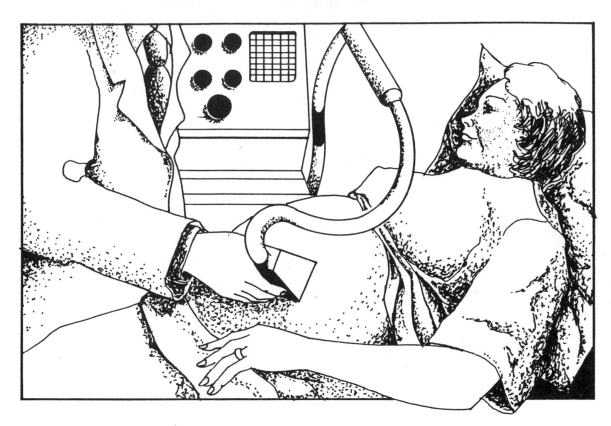

More About Pregnancy

L abor and delivery—finally, the moment arrives when all the work you have done to keep you and your baby healthy becomes all worth it. For most women, the birth of their baby is an exhilarating, joyful experience. Of course, labor itself is not fun and it is natural for you to be a little scared or apprehensive about delivering your baby. However, because of the technology we have to monitor your health and that of your baby, the chances for a successful pregnancy are now better than ever.

So, relax. Take a deep breath. Let it out slowly. Turn the page and focus your thoughts on the next chapters.

Tests To Expect During Your Pregnancy 8

During your pregnancy, you will probably go through several different types of tests, technically known as *antepartum* testing. (Antepartum means before labor or childbirth.) In general, antepartum testing is divided into two categories. In the first category are those tests given during the first half of pregnancy, called *diagnostic prenatal testing*. These tests are intended to detect structural or genetic disorders in your developing baby. The second category of tests is started later in pregnancy, usually in the third trimester, and these tests are often continued until delivery. These tests are called *fetal surveillance*. Some of these tests measure your baby's growth. Others evaluate the condition of your baby. This is done by checking how well the placenta supplies your baby with oxygen and nutrients. Here are tests that you may experience during your pregnancy:

Diagnostic Prenatal Testing

Serum Alpha Fetoprotein (AFP) During the first part of the second trimester (around 16 weeks from your last menstrual period), an AFP test may be ordered. This test measures the level of AFP in *your* blood and looks for *neural tube* defects such as *spina bifida* or *anencephaly*. (The neural tube is the initial organ from which your baby's brain and spinal cord develop. Spina bifida is a defect in the spinal cord. With anencephaly the brain does not develop fully.) The risk for these defects is quite low. Among women with diabetes, only 6 to 8 per 1,000 will have a baby with neural tube defects, and serum AFP testing will identify 75 percent of these pregnancies.

The AFP test is a *screening* test which identifies those pregnancies that are at risk but does not make a specific diagnosis. In other words, this test tells you something is not right, but it cannot tell what exactly is wrong. Many factors other than a neural tube defect can cause the AFP level to be abnormal. In fact, 5 of each 100 women tested will have an abnormal test value. When this happens, other diagnostic procedures, such as ultrasound or amniocentesis, are used. Many women whose test results show abnormal values go on to deliver perfectly healthy babies.

Diagnostic Prenatal Testing

- **Serum Alpha Fetoprotein (AFP)**
- **Ultrasound**
- **Genetic Counseling and Testing**

Ultrasound   Ultrasound tests use sound waves to outline and photograph organs—including a developing baby—inside the human body. The picture that is taken is called a *sonogram*. This procedure has been used for about 20 years, and studies have not revealed any harmful effects to mothers or their babies.

Before the test, you may be asked to drink lots of fluids. So that your bladder will be full, you will also be asked not to urinate. This allows the person doing the test to make certain measurements more easily.

The procedure uses a machine with a monitor screen to produce the pictures. The testing is painless. You lie on your back while a moveable arm or probe (called a *transducer*) is gently glided across your abdomen. Ultrasound testing identifies the number of babies, their position in the uterus, and the outline and structure of their bodies. Ultrasound is usually performed in the second half of pregnancy. By this time, the baby is large enough for all the distinct features to show up on the test. It can sometimes detect the sex of your baby, though sex determinations are not always accurate. It also helps in estimating how far along your pregnancy is. However, it is not always possible to identify birth defects with a sonogram.

Because you have diabetes, your baby may be larger or smaller than average. Ultrasound is often repeated at monthly intervals to determine your baby's rate of growth.

Genetic counseling and testing   Just because you have diabetes does not mean you are automatically more at a risk for giving birth to a baby with genetic disorders. However, other factors—unrelated to diabetes—may present an increased risk for genetic problems in your baby. For example, when the mother is 35 years or older, the risk of genetic disorders increases. A previous family history of genetic disorders is also a factor. Some common genetic disorders are cystic fibrosis, muscular dystrophy, and Down's syndrome.

If you are at risk for having a baby with genetic disorders, you may be referred for genetic counseling. This includes an evaluation and explanation of your specific risk for delivering a child with a particular genetic disorder. Testing options, including the risks of the procedures, will be explained.

The most common type of genetic testing is a procedure called *amniocentesis*, which is usually done around the fourth month of pregnancy. It is performed by taking a sample of amniotic fluid that surrounds the baby (the bag of waters).

When amniocentesis is performed, ultrasound is used to find the baby and the best "pocket" of fluid. A needle is then inserted through the mother's abdomen to remove a small amount (usually less than an ounce) of the fluid, which is then tested in a laboratory to make a diagnosis. Most of the time, this test is done by growing some of the cells (a tissue culture) that were floating around in the fluid. Growing the tissue culture takes weeks. Experts then examine the tissue culture to determine the genetic structure.

Waiting for these test results and the results themselves may be emotionally difficult for you and your partner. The decisions you and your partner may have to make, as a result of these tests, could also be difficult. For this reason, you should receive as much information as possible about your particular risks and the options available to you.

Some decisions you make about yourself and your family are very difficult, but *only you* can make them. Being informed is vital. Your health-care team is available to provide emotional support when you need it.

Fetal Surveillance

A number of methods to evaluate the health of a developing baby have been devised over the years. No method is clearly superior to the others—different centers caring for high-risk pregnancies vary in their choice of tests. It is best to use the test (or tests) that a particular center is most familiar and comfortable with. This is fine since all methods are designed to provide similar information about your developing baby's health. The commonly used tests will be described here. You may be tested with one or more of the following:

Kick counts   The movements or kicks that you feel from your baby are one important indicator of your baby's health. You may be asked to count the number of times you feel your baby move during a particular time each day. Your doctor or nurse/educator will explain how and when to do these counts and will also explain how to recognize serious problems and when to alert your health-care practitioner. In general, when you detect a change in the pattern of your baby's movement, you should notify your health-care team—they may want to do further testing.

Contraction Stress Test (CST)   This test measures how well the placenta transfers oxygen from you to your baby. This test is performed by attaching an electronic *fetal monitor* to your abdomen. This monitor prints out, on a strip of paper, your baby's heart rate and the contractions of your uterus. If you are having frequent contractions (even though you may not actually be in labor), the response of your baby's heart to the stress of each contraction indicates the health of your baby and the placenta. If you are not having contractions, an intravenous (IV) line may be placed in your arm, and you will

Fetal Surveillance

- **Kick Count**
- **Contraction Stress Test (CST)**
- **Non-Stress Test (NST)**
- **Biophysical Profile (BPP)**
- **Amniocentesis**

be given a medication called *oxytocin (Pitocin)*, which causes you to have contractions. This test, called an *oxytocin challenge test* (OCT), usually takes 60 to 90 minutes.

Non-Stress Test (NST)   This test is also used to determine the state of your baby and the placenta. Just as in the CST, the fetal monitor is placed on your abdomen. However, this test measures changes in your baby's heart rate when he or she kicks—not the heart-rate response to contractions in your uterus. This test checks the acceleration (speeding up) of your baby's heart rate at times of activity. This acceleration suggests that your baby is healthy. The test is painless and usually takes 30 to 45 minutes and can be performed in your doctor's office.

Biophysical Profile (BPP)   In this test, ultrasound is used to evaluate your baby's movement, body tone, breathing, and the amount of amniotic fluid surrounding your baby. (Although no air is in your uterus, your baby does make breathing motions while inside you. Amniotic fluid is drawn in and out of the lungs.)

Amniocentesis   This procedure was discussed on page 48 under diagnostic prenatal testing; however, it is also useful in fetal surveillance. Amniocentesis helps determine when it is safe to deliver your baby. Sometimes it is necessary to induce labor or deliver a baby by cesarean section (see page 51). Before either procedure is performed, it may be necessary to find out whether your baby's lungs are mature. If your baby is delivered before the lungs are mature, a problem called *respiratory distress syndrome* may make it difficult for your newborn to breathe normally. By doing an amniocentesis to obtain amniotic fluid, a test can be done to see if your baby's lungs are mature enough to breathe on their own. This test will help predict whether respiratory distress syndrome is likely. The actual procedure is exactly the same as that described earlier, but the results of the test are usually available within 24 hours.

CHAPTER 9

Labor and Delivery

Before we knew the techniques for tight control of blood glucose, the risks for giving birth to a very large baby or for having a stillbirth were quite high. In the past, a woman with diabetes was usually admitted to the hospital during the final weeks of pregnancy, and delivery was induced early.

Now that self-monitoring of blood glucose is possible, most women with diabetes can remain safely home until labor begins. And they can have their babies on or near their due dates. Hence, fewer premature babies are born to women who have diabetes. (Premature babies may have immature lungs and have trouble breathing after delivery.)

After studying your health and that of your baby, and how your pregnancy is progressing, your health-care team will determine the best time and mode of delivery for both you and your baby. It's possible that your labor will start on its own and your baby will be born vaginally (through the vagina). If your labor does not start on its own, it may be induced with a hormone called *oxytocin*. Oxytocin speeds up labor by causing the uterine muscles to contract. If you can't deliver your baby vaginally or if there is a problem, then you will need to have your baby by an operation called a cesarean section (C-section), or cesarean birth.

During a C-section, an incision is made through the abdomen and uterus, through which the baby is removed. Because of the surgery, your recovery may be longer than if you delivered your baby vaginally. Generally, a woman who has a C-section needs to stay in the hospital four to five days and takes four to six weeks to fully recover.

Many babies born to women with diabetes are delivered by a C-section. The reason may be because many give birth to large babies who cannot fit through the birth canal.

However, the size of your baby is not the only reason a C-section may be necessary. In some cases, labor can be stressful for a baby, and a C-section may be necessary to ensure the baby's health. If you've had a C-section before, you may choose to deliver future babies this way. Finally, health complications may make a C-section necessary. Be sure to discuss a C-section with your health-care team months before your baby is born. It's best for you to be prepared for whatever may happen.

To determine the safest time and method to deliver your baby, your health-care team will examine a variety of factors: blood-glucose control, blood pressure, kidney function, and diabetes complications. The team will also study your baby's size and movements, his or her heart-rate pattern, and the amount of amniotic fluid in the uterus.

In some cases, a small amount of fluid will be withdrawn from your uterus (see amniocentesis, page 48). This procedure will help determine whether your baby's lungs are mature and help guide the timing of delivery. While you are in labor, your baby's heart rate and well-being will probably be monitored by a *fetal monitor*.

Keeping your blood-glucose level as normal as possible will be a major concern during your labor and delivery, regardless of when or how your baby is delivered. Your having a normal glucose level during labor and delivery will reduce the risk of your baby having low blood glucose after delivery. Remember, if your blood glucose is high, the glucose crosses the placenta and may cause your baby's pancreas to produce too much insulin.

In general, labor, like any strenuous exercise, tends to lower blood glucose in a person whose diabetes is well-controlled. So, you will probably need less insulin during active labor. Your blood glucose will be checked frequently (probably every few hours) and your insulin and glucose regimen will be tailored to your needs during this time.

It's obvious that you want to be prepared by knowing what you can about your pregnancy and the birth of your baby. That you're reading this book demonstrates your interest. To help you prepare for labor, many hospitals and other organizations offer classes (such as Lamaze) to help you have a smooth delivery. They teach you what to expect during labor, techniques to improve delivery and to relieve pain during labor, and how to care for your baby after birth. If you're interested in such a class, ask your doctor or check with your hospital about classes in your area.

Finally, we want to add this warning: Some women desire to give birth in the home. However, because of the care needed to perform a successful delivery, home births are not recommended for women who have diabetes.

Lactation

Nearly all women are encouraged to breast-feed their babies. Breast milk is healthy for the baby: It contains antibodies to fight certain infections. Breast milk has other advantages, too—it is readily available, inexpensive, and convenient. In

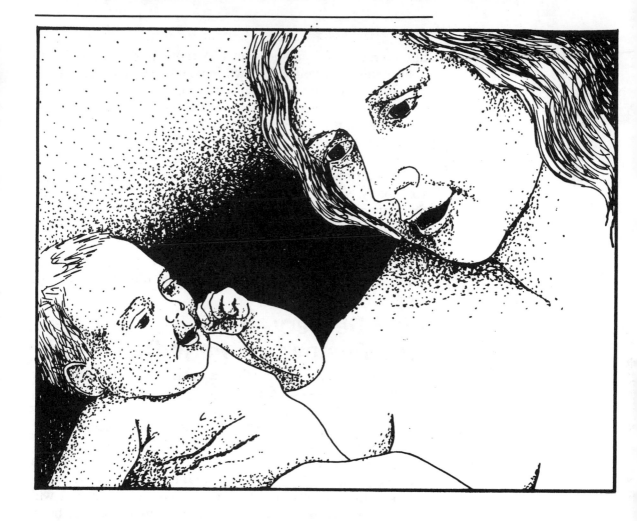

addition, breast-feeding will help you bond with your baby. Breast-feeding can also help you lose some of the weight you gained during pregnancy. It might even prove a good way to help you lose any excess fat you had before you were pregnant.

Most women lose between 12 and 15 pounds during the first week after giving birth. The total weight you gained during pregnancy should be gradually lost over a three-month period. If your health-care practitioner recommends that you lose weight, you can begin during the time you are breast-feeding. However, you should generally wait two to four weeks after your baby's birth before you begin to lose this weight.

During the time that you breast-feed, you need to pay close attention to what you eat. The same meal plan you had before you were pregnant should cover the demands of breast-feeding. If you are in doubt, check with your dietitian to find a meal plan to meet your needs.

While you are breast-feeding, it is important that you get the right amounts of calcium, fluids, and protein. Breast milk is amazingly constant in composition, but the quantity of milk changes depending on how much fluid you drink. If you reduce the amount of food that you eat, the quantity of your milk will also be reduced. You and your dietitian can discuss and plan your meals to fit your needs while you are breast-feeding.

Breast-feeding may also require insulin adjustments, especially in your overnight dosage. This is because your blood-glucose level may drop while you are breast-feeding and you can lose glucose during your baby's bedtime and late-night feedings. Ask how to make these adjustments.

While breast-feeding may be a perfect way to nourish your baby, you may be unable or unwilling to breast-feed. Some women are uncomfortable breast-feeding. Some have full-time jobs that make breast-feeding on a regular schedule difficult. Others, because of health reasons, are unable to breast-feed. If you can't or don't want to breast-feed, don't feel guilty. Your baby will still do well and get the nutrients he or she needs from a formula.

After Delivery (The Postpartum Period)

Soon after you give birth, major changes will occur. Your weight and level of activity will change during this time. Also, you may experience emotional ups and downs—many new mothers do. After your baby is born, your insulin needs will be much less than they were during your pregnancy.

For a short time, your insulin needs may even be less than they were before you became pregnant. Blood-glucose monitoring is the best way to chart these rapid changes and will make it easier to make the necessary adjustments as your body returns to its *nonpregnant* state. A few weeks after delivery, your insulin dose should return to the level it was before you became pregnant.

If you didn't take control of your diabetes before you were pregnant, you probably learned a great deal from taking control during your pregnancy. Now that you're in the habit, it will be easier to continue practicing good control. You'll be happy you did—and so will your new family.

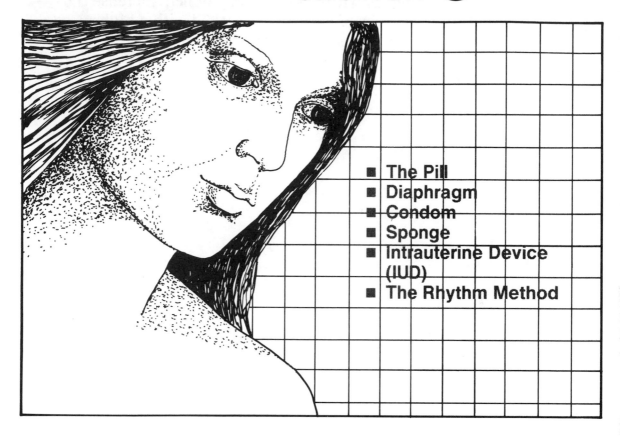

- The Pill
- Diaphragm
- Condom
- Sponge
- Intrauterine Device (IUD)
- The Rhythm Method

Birth Control

Some women may wonder what a section on birth control is doing in a book about pregnancy. Many of you may think it's a little late to be talking about that now. However, there are a couple reasons for this section. First, this book is not just for the woman who *is* pregnant, but also for the woman who is *thinking* about having a baby. She needs to consider birth control until she is ready to have a baby. Second, after a woman has a baby, birth control is important.

There are many options on the market today and it is important that you and your partner consider each one. Some methods of birth control may work better and fit into your lifestyle more

easily. Some are safer for you than others. Making
an informed choice, which includes discussing birth
control with your doctor, will help increase the
chances of choosing a method with a high success
rate, and one with fewer health risks to you.

Making 10
The Choice

Choosing the safest and most appropriate time to have a child is one of the keys to planning a successful pregnancy for a woman with diabetes. Of course, *planning* a pregnancy means that you are going to use some form of birth control (contraception) until you are ready to try to have a baby.

Many women with diabetes are concerned about the safety of various methods of contraception, the advantages and disadvantages of each, and whether one method is better than the others. One of the most important aspects of family planning is choosing the right method of birth control for *you* and your partner.

A number of different methods are available and no one method is right for *all* individuals. You have special needs that may make one form of birth control better for you than another. The important factor in choosing any method is that it should be reliable and effective. Unfortunately, not all the methods available today offer the protection you need. It is important that you and your partner discuss and find a birth control method that suits both of you. Here are some of the birth control methods being used today:

The Pill Oral contraception, or the birth control pill, is one of the most popular methods of birth control. However, popularity doesn't mean the pill's the best for you. The advantage of birth control pills is their reliability. They are 99 percent effective *when taken as directed*.

There are two types of birth control pills: the combination pill, which contains estrogen and progestogen (sex hormones), and the progestogen-only pill. The combination pill is believed to be slightly more effective than the progestogen-only pill: 99 percent versus 98 percent. The progestogen-only pill can also cause irregular bleeding and weight gain.

In women with insulin-dependent diabetes, the combination pill can interfere with diabetes control. So, if you go on the pill, you will probably have to increase the amount of insulin you inject. The short-term risks (a year or two) are slight, but scientists are not certain about the risks of using the pill for longer periods of time. If you develop high blood pressure while taking the pill, this could increase the risk that retinopathy or kidney disease will progress. Because of this, you need to know if you have any complications before you start using birth control pills. And you and your health-care practitioner need to discuss your specific risks for using the pill.

Diaphragm   The diaphragm is a rubber cap that the woman lubricates with a spermicidal gel and inserts into her vagina before intercourse. It fits over the cervix and acts as a barrier to prevent sperm from entering the cervix and passing to the uterus. The uterus is where the eggs are fertilized by the sperm. For this reason, the diaphragm is called a *barrier method* of birth control. When used correctly, it can be up to 95 percent effective in preventing pregnancy.

Some women find a diaphragm awkward and difficult to use. And they fear it affects the spontaneity of lovemaking. It is true that using a diaphragm won't be the same as going without. But, because the diaphragm can be inserted as much as an hour before intercourse, a little planning ahead will allow you to have some level of spontaneity. If you choose a diaphragm, it is important that you have your doctor make sure the diaphragm fits you properly. Also, make sure he or she explains how to use it correctly. Many doctors recommend the diaphragm for women with diabetes.

Condom   Another barrier method of birth control is the condom, a thin membrane sheath that fits over the penis. It can be used effectively by itself, but it is even more effective when combined with a sperm-killing foam or vaginal gel suppository. Statistics indicate that when the condom and foam are used together, they are up to 85 percent effective in preventing pregnancy.

The major problem with barrier methods of birth control, such as the condom, is that they require some planning for use. They must be used every time intercourse occurs, and they must be used correctly. If not, they won't be as effective.

Sponge   This is a small sponge-like object that contains a sperm-killing gel. The sponge is placed in the vagina before intercourse. Researchers have not determined how reliable the sponge is in preventing pregnancy. Therefore, the sponge is not recommended.

Intrauterine Device (IUD)   An IUD is a small plastic device that is placed inside the uterus by a physician. Some IUDs were suspected to cause pelvic infections in women who used them and were taken off the market. Because they have been linked with infections, IUDs are not generally recommended for women who have diabetes. You should discuss with your doctor or health-care practitioner any benefits or risks involved in your using an IUD.

The Rhythm Method The least effective method of birth control is the rhythm method. This method is one of the oldest types of birth control, but unfortunately, it is not effective. The rhythm method requires the most effort of all birth control methods. In general, it works by avoiding intercourse 3 to 4 days around the time you ovulate. Unfortunately, this method is much more complicated—you have to know exactly when you ovulate.

Most women ovulate during the middle of their menstrual periods, but menstrual cycles can be irregular so it can be difficult to determine the exact time of ovulation. The best, yet still inaccurate, method of trying to determine when you ovulate is to measure your rectal temperature. This is because body temperature changes slightly at the time of ovulation. To be as accurate as possible, you need to check your temperature *daily* in the early morning *before* you get out of bed. This method requires a lot of planning to make it even somewhat successful. Therefore, it is not recommended for women with diabetes.

Finally, while we are on the subject of birth control, you may wonder how soon after giving birth you can have intercourse. Unfortunately, there are no absolute answers to this important question. It is probably a good idea to wait at least three or four weeks to give the muscles in the walls of your vagina time to strengthen. And if you had an episiotomy, it will have time to heal. (An episiotomy is an incision made between the vagina and anus to help keep that area from tearing during the vaginal birth of your baby.) Check with your doctor to see how long he or she suggests you wait.

Also, remember that you could become pregnant soon after you give birth. Even if you have not had a menstrual period, you still may ovulate. Also, breast-feeding your baby *will not* prevent you from becoming pregnant.

Choosing birth control is a personal matter—the decision is up to you. Be sure to discuss the different types of birth control with your health-care practitioner. The more information you have, the better you can make a decision that will be best for you.

Conclusion

As you can see, the success of your pregnancy depends a lot on how well you take control of your diabetes. At first, controlling your diabetes during pregnancy may seem impossible. It is normal for you to feel that way, but you can do it! True, controlling your diabetes during pregnancy won't be easy—it *will* take time and it *will* take dedication. The important thing to remember is that you have help. Your health-care team will help you make the adjustments you need to keep your diabetes in control during this very special time.

Of course, the most important thing to remember is the end result—a happy, healthy, beautiful baby. Once that baby is born, we're sure you'll agree that the time you took to control your diabetes was well worth it!

Glossary

Abruption (ablatio placentae): Separation of the placenta from the uterus while the fetus is in utero. It can be life-threatening for the baby and requires emergency medical treatment.

Amniocentesis: Puncture of the amniotic sac (bag of waters) with a needle to obtain a sample of fluid for examination.

Carbohydrate: A class of food that is either a simple or a complex starch that the body breaks into simple sugar once it is eaten.

Contraction Stress Test (CST): A test in which a hormone is given to cause the uterus to contract. The baby's heart rate is monitored during this test.

Dietitian: Also known as a Nutritionist. A specialist in food and diet.

Endocrinologist: A physician who specializes in glandular diseases. Diabetes is a disease of the gland called the pancreas.

Gestational Diabetes (GDM): Diabetes that occurs during pregnancy and goes away after pregnancy. GDM is diagnosed based on a standard glucose tolerance test.

Glucose: A simple sugar.

Hyperbilirubinemia: Elevation of bilirubin above normal.

Hyperglycemia: Blood glucose levels above normal. If left untreated, can lead to coma and death.

Hypoglycemia: Blood glucose levels below normal which can result in sweating, irritability, shakiness, a fast pulse, or unconsciousness if not corrected.

Insulin: The hormone necessary to help the body use and/or store sugar.

Ketosis: Breakdown of body fat into acids that occurs when the body does not have enough food or enough insulin.

Lethargic: Very sleepy.

Neonatologist: A pediatrician who specializes in caring for newborn infants.

Non-stress Test (NST): Monitoring of the baby's heart rate (pulse) when he or she kicks.

Obstetrician: A physician who specializes in caring for pregnant women.

Oxytocin: The hormone that causes the womb to contract.

Pancreas: The organ in the body that produces the hormone insulin.

Pediatrician: A physician who specializes in caring for children.

Placenta: The organ between mother and baby that allows nutrients and sugar from the mother to be passed freely into the baby's bloodstream, but does not allow insulin to pass.

Prematurity: Birth before the baby is mature.

Sonogram: A sound wave picture of the baby.

Stillbirth: The death of an unborn child. Technically this term is reserved for unborn children more than halfway along in the womb.

Uterus: Womb.

INDEX

For More Information

The American Diabetes Association (ADA) is the nation's leading voluntary health organization dedicated to improving the well-being of all people with diabetes and their families. Equally important is our unceasing support for research to find a preventive and cure for this chronic disease, which affects some 14 million Americans. The American Diabetes Association provides information and support for those who have the disease, and educates health-care professionals and the general public about the seriousness of diabetes. The Association carries out this important mission through the efforts of thousands of volunteers working at affiliates and chapters in more than 800 communities across the United States.

ADA membership puts you in contact with a network of more than 270,000 caring people in communities like yours. Our local affiliates and chapters offer services you can't find anywhere else, such as support groups, educational programs, counseling, and special camps for kids with diabetes. In addition, we publish a variety of materials for people of every age group on topics of importance not only to the individual with diabetes but to the entire family as well. Membership in your local ADA affiliate carries with it many benefits, including a subscription to *Diabetes Forecast*, our lively patient education magazine, published monthly. The American Diabetes Association also distributes a free quarterly newsletter. To obtain membership information or to order the newsletter, contact the Association at the address below. To find your local affiliate, look in the white pages of your phone directory, or contact:

American Diabetes Association®, Inc.
Diabetes Information Service Center
1660 Duke Street
Alexandria, VA 22314
Tel: 800-232-3472

Other Publications

Delicious, Nutritional Cooking

All of ADA's cookbooks have specially developed, kitchen-tested recipes, and each volume has a completely different set of delicious menu suggestions. Each volume also has a special nutrients-per-serving breakdown for each recipe, plus exchange values based on the *Exchange Lists for Meal Planning*.

Family Cookbook, Volume I

More than 250 delicious, economical, kitchen-tested recipes fill the pages of Volume I. It offers an encyclopedia of nutrition information, tips on eating out, brown-bagging, weight control, exercise and much more. 1987. 388 pages. Hardcover. #CCBF1
Member: $17.95   **Nonmember:** $19.95

Family Cookbook, Volume II

Volume II includes ways to cut sugar, calories, and costs—plus there are more than 250 tasty recipes! It has an entire section devoted to living with diabetes and gives advice on the emotional aspects of dieting. 1987. 452 pages. Hardcover. #CCBF2
Member: $20.70   **Nonmember:** $23.00

Family Cookbook, Volume III

Add to your recipe treasury with more than 200 delicious recipes. Included are tips on microwaving, food processing, and freezing for fix-ahead meals. Recipes from various ethnic cuisines are included. 1987. 434 pages. Hardcover. #CCBF3
Member: $20.70   **Nonmember:** $23.00

Brand New!
Family Cookbook, Volume IV

Recipes from Boston Scrod to Santa Fe Chicken (more than 200 recipes in all) fill each page of this new cookbook with great American flavor. *Family Cookbook, Vol. IV* also includes a colorful section of interesting facts about the history of American cuisine. 1991. 403 pages. Hardcover. #CCBF4
Member: $20.70   **Nonmember:** $23.00

American Diabetes Association
Holiday Cookbook
by Betty Wedman, M.S., R.D.
Enjoy the holidays more with recipes from traditional Thanksgiving, Christmas, and Hanukkah feasts . . . to savory meals for any occasion. 1986. 219 pages. Hardcover. #CCBH
Member: $17.95   **Nonmember:** $19.95

American Diabetes Association Special Celebrations and Parties Cookbook
by Betty Wedman, M.S., R.D.
Whether it's a Fourth of July barbecue, Mother's Day brunch, or birthday bash, these recipes invite everyone to join in. 1989. 256 pages. Hardcover. #CCBSCP
Member: $17.95   **Nonmember:** $19.95

Healthy Eating

Exchange Lists for Meal Planning
Colorful charts, helpful tips on good nutrition, and the six easy-to-use food Exchange Lists show you how to balance your diet and gain control over diabetes. 1989. 32 pages. Softcover. #CELMP
Member: $1.10   **Nonmember:** $1.30

Eating Healthy Foods
This booklet provides daily food choices for breakfast, lunch, dinner, and snacks using the Exchange Lists. 1988. 16 pages. Softcover. #CELEHF
Member: $1.70   **Nonmember:** $2.00

Month of Meals
Choose from 28 days' worth of breakfasts, lunches, and dinners that figure your calories and exchanges for you. There's also a selection of delicious snacks and many of the menus have recipes, too! 1989. 57 pages. Spiral-bound. #CMPMOM
Member: $9.00   **Nonmember:** $10.00

Month of Meals 2
Another menu-planning book that can help you decide what to eat and how to fix it! You get 28 days' worth of new breakfast, lunch, and dinner choices, plus tips on dining out at Mexican, Italian, Chinese, and fast food restaurants. 1990. 64 pages. Spiral-bound. #CMPMOM2
Member: $9.00   **Non-member:** $10.00

Brand New!
Month of Meals 3
Breakfast, lunch, and dinner choices continue to grow with Month of Meals 3. Special sections include: how to read ingredient labels on packages; how to have picnics & barbecues and stay within your meal plan; more! 1992. Spiral-bound. #CMPMOM3
Member: $9.00   **Non-member:** $10.00

To Order ADA Publications
Send your check or money order payable to:
American Diabetes Association
1970 Chain Bridge Road
McLean, VA 22109-0592

Allow 4–6 weeks for delivery. Add $3.00 to shipping & handling for each additional "ship to" address. Foreign orders must be paid in U.S. funds, drawn on a U.S. bank. Prices subject to change without notice.

Shipping & Handling Chart:
up to $5.00 .... add **$1.75**
$5.01–$10.00 .... add **$3.00**
$10.01–$25.00 .... add **$4.50**
$25.01–$50.00 .... add **$5.50**
over $50.00 .... add **10% of order**